# Cannabis Oil Cures

*How to cure cancer for life, improve health immediately, lose weight within 30 days and look younger with Cannabis Oil*

# Table of Contents

# Introduction

I want to thank you and congratulate you for purchasing this book.

In the mid 70s, scientist became aware of the many beneficial effects of cannabinoid compounds over cancerous cell. Over the past ten years, more than a dozen medical studies have revealed how cancer can be cured with these cannabinoid compounds. However, big pharma companies are still opposing the cancer cure and keep endorsing chemotherapy and their own lineup of harmful drugs to doctors and patients.

Laboratory tests conducted in 2008 by an international team of scientists and published in The Journal Of Clinical Investigation, revealed that the active ingredient in marijuana, labeled as tetrahydrocannabinol or THC, can function as a cure for brain cancer by inducing human glioma cell death through stimulation of autophagy.

The study determined that THC can terminate multiple types of cancers, affecting various cells in the body. Other studies have revealed that cannabinoids may also inhibit cell growth, induce cell death, and inhibit tumor metastasis.

What is astounding is that, unlike chemotherapy, cannabinoids effectively target and kill cancerous cells, and do not affect healthy, normal cells. Cannabinoids actually protect healthy cells against cellular death.

Cannabinoids are also researched for their pain-modulation and anti-inflammatory abilities as they bind to special receptors in the brain, much like opioid derivatives that are commonly prescribed today.

Further evidence to support the effects of cannabis extract on malignant cells comes from the real life experience of individuals who have successfully overcome cancer by using cannabis oil.

What stands out is that from the vast amount of research and data available, as well as the personal experiences of cancer survivors, is that no chemotherapy currently being used medically can match the non-toxic anti-carcinogenic and anti-tumorigenic effects of these natural plant compounds.

The following pages will discuss Cannabis Oil, its safety in topical and oral use, its different medical uses, how to properly dose and apply it, and how to make your own Cannabis oil. Additionally, you will find real life examples of people who have used Cannabis Oil to cure cancer, improved their overall health and live a rejuvenated life.

# Chapter 1: How Cannabis Oil Works

In order to understand how cannabis oil fights cancer cells, it is important to first understand what sustains the existence of cancer cells in the body. Once this is understood, we will proceed to examining how cannabidiol (cannabinoids CBD) and tetrahydrocannabino (THC), two components found in cannabis, eliminate cancer cells.

While the following paragraphs may seem very technical, I recommend that you read them slowly and carefully in order to fully grasp the powerful healing attributes provided by the use of cannabis. So here we go.

Each of our cells contains a group of inter-convertible sphingolipids, which control the life and death of the cells. The overall term of the various factors that comprise this is referred to as "Sphingolipid Rheostat". Endogenous ceramide is sphingosine-1 phosphate's signaling metabolite. If high levels of endogenous ceramide occur in the cell, its death is forthcoming. When cells have low level in, it means that the cell has robust vitality.

To put it in simpler terms, when THC attaches itself to the so-called CB2 or CB1 cannabinoid receptor sites on the cancerous cells, it causes accelerated ceramide synthesis, which in turn accelerates the death of the cells. When THC is present in the cells, the cells do not generate ceramide as it is normal and healthy. This means that with THC occurring in the cells, the cells are not disturbed by the cannabinoid.

The death of the cancer cell does not actually result from cytotoxic chemicals but from the minuscule changes in the mitochondria, the "powerhouses of the cell". The majority of our body's cells is composed of a cell nucleus, hundreds or thousands of mitochondria and other different organelles in the cytoplasm. The main function of the mitochondria is to generate ATP or energy to be used by the cells. When ceramide is accumulated in the cell, it turns up the Sphingolipid Rheostat which in turn intensifies the permeability of cytochrome c in the mitochondrial membrane pores, essentially forcing them out. Cytochrome c is a vital protein required for the synthesis of energy. When cytochrome c is eliminated out of the mitochondria, the cell's energy source is killed.

Ceramide also causes genotoxic stress in the cancerous cell nucleus. This then leads to the generation of p53, which is a protein that is responsible for the disruption of calcium metabolism in the mitochondria. In addition, ceramide also causes the disruption of the cellular lysosome, which functions as the digestive system of the cells that supplies the nutrients required by the cells in order to function properly.

To sum it up, when ceramide and other sphingolipids are present, pro-survival pathways in the cells are actively inhibited, which makes it utterly impossible for the cancer cells to survive.

The basis of this process is the ceramide buildup in the system. This means that when you take therapeutic amounts of THC and CBD on a regular basis over an extended period of time, you can keep enough metabolic pressure on the death pathway of the cancer cells.

Here is where cannabis oil comes into the picture. You may wonder how the human body can receive a simple plant enzyme and utilize it for the intense restoration and treatment in various physiological systems. How can it provide both palliative and curative properties? How can one plant be so safe while at the same time offering highly powerful effects? To answer these questions, scientists have led extensive research projects and eventually discovered a formerly unknown physiologic system, which plays a central role in health and healing of every human and almost every animal: the endocannabinoid system, called after the plant that led to its discovery. This endogenous cannabinoid system is thought to be the most significant physiological system involved in regulating and preserving human health. Endocannabinoids and their receptors are found within the whole body, such as the brain, organs, glands, connective tissue and immune cells. The cannabinoid system has different responsibilities in each tissue, but the overall goal is always the same: homeostasis, which is the maintenance of a stable internal environment while adjusting to conditions that are optimal for survival.

One example of cannabinoids creating homeostasis is autophagy, a process that degrades and digests unnecessary, or feeble and dysfunctional components within the cell. While this mechanism keeps healthy cells alive, it has a deadly effect on unhealthy, abnormal cells, such as malignant tumor cells, causing them to consume themselves in a programmed cellular suicide. Eliminating cancer cells causes homeostasis, the perfect balance and survival of the organism.

How cannabinoids work at the cellular level:

The endocannabinoids originate directly from the brain's synapses. When the body is compromised because of an injury or illness, it immediately activates the endocannabinoid system and orders the immune system to start the healing process. If the homeostatic system of the body is damaged because of cancer, the intake of exocannabinoid can help the body by doing the job of endocannabinoid system in the most natural way possible.

In order to better understand the process, you can imagine the cannabinoid as a molecule with three dimensions wherein each part or dimension of the molecule is designed to match the immune or nerve cell receptor site similar to how a key matches a lock. At the minimum, there are two kinds of cannabinoid receptor sites - CB1 for the central nervous system (CNS) and CB2 for the immune system. Generally, CB1 triggers the messaging system of the CNS while CB2 triggers the messaging system of the immune system.

But the process is not really that simple. Both anandamide and THC can also trigger the two receptor sites. There are also other cannabinoids that can trigger any of the receptor sites. Cannabis sativa has the tendency to activate the CB1 receptor while Cannabis indica has the tendency to activate the CB2 receptor. This means that C. indica is more immuno-active while C. sativa is more neuro-active. You also need to consider the fact that C. sativa is controlled by THC cannabinoids while C. indica is predominantly CBD.

Research studies have shown that CBD and THC are biomimetic to anandamide. This means that the human body can utilize both CBD and THC interchangeably. When your body has an illness or is injured or stressed out, it demands more endogenous anandamide than your body can produce. As such, the mimetic exocannabinoids are triggered to produce the anandamide. If the stress to your body is temporary, the treatment required is also temporary. But if the higher demand is persistent, such as with cancer, the treatment should be able to supply continued pressure of the modulating agent on the various homeostatic systems.

Normally CBD is drawn to the tightly packed CB2 receptors in the spleen which is considered as the base of the immune system of the body. When CBD reaches the spleen, immune cells will start to search for and abolish the cancer cells. Remarkably, research studies show that CBD and THC cannabinoids have the capability to directly abolish cancer cells without the need to go through any of the immune intermediaries. CBD and THC take over the control of the lipoxygenase pathway and immediately prevent the growth of the tumor. This means that cannabidiol aids the body in preserving its own natural endocannabinoid by preventing the spread of the enzyme that causes anandamide breakdown.

This goes to show that nature has created the perfect remedy that exactly matches the receptors of the immune system of the human body and signals metabolites to supply complete and fast immune response for metabolic homeostasis and systemic integrity.

# Chapter 2: How to Make Your Own Cannabis Oil

Cannabis oil, sometimes also referred to as RSO, marijuana oil, Rick Simpson Oil, weed oil, hash oil and pot oil is highly effective way to use for your treatment of cancer and various other diseases. To make your own cannabis oil at home, please carefully follow the instructions below. There are various methods for making cannabis oil, however this chapter will focus on the easiest method, which will allow you to produce cannabis oil using the supplies that are usually available at home.

1. Note on the materials needed

To begin the treatment of most cancers, you will require around 60 g/ml of cannabis oil. To make a full treatment of 60 g/ml, you will require one or more pounds of high grade cannabis and two gallons of solvent. It is ideal to look for the driest cannabis that you can find. But if you do not really wish to make a full treatment, you can make cannabis oil with a minimum of 1 ounce of cannabis. With each ounce of high quality cannabis bud, you can normally produce around 3 to 5 grams of cannabis oil. The actual quantity of oil that you can produce for each ounce of cannabis will depend on the specific type of strain of the cannabis. But no matter what strain you choose, all of them have remarkable healing powers.

For the solvent, it is ideal to use 190 proof Ever-clear alcohol or 99% to 100% isopropyl alcohol. DO NOT use VM&P naptha, Coleman fuel or heavy naptha because those solvents can result in residual solvent in your cannabis oil. You need to keep in mind that producing cannabis oil can be hazardous especially if you do not take proper safeguards and precautions. Make sure that you are wearing suitable safety equipment such as gloves, safety masks or safety glasses before starting the production to lessen your contact to the solvent. It is also vital that your fan is turned on while working to help in carrying the vapors of the solvent away. When you do not use a fan, the solvent can form a puddle beneath the rice cooker which is very hazardous. Remember, extreme caution should be your number one priority when making cannabis oil.

2. Materials Needed:

- Odor respirator or paint mask

- Electric candle warmer

- Non-latex safety gloves

- Box fan or table fan

- High heat gloves or oven mitts

- Thermometer

- Safety glasses

- Electric rice cooker

- Large funnel

- 190 proof Everclear alcohol or 99% to 100% isopropyl alcohol

- Large stainless steel bowls

- Coffee filters

- Large bottles for holding solvent-oil mixture

- High temp silicone scraper set

- Stainless measuring cups

- Wooden or stainless cooking spoons

- Pyrex storage dish

- Stainless mesh strainer

Directions:

1. Put the cannabis in a container that is large enough to allow mixing.

2. Wash the cannabis material using your preferred solvent. You will need around 2 gallons of solvent to remove all the THC and other cannabinoids from 1 lb. of dry cannabis material.

3. Gently crush the dampened cannabis. This action dissolves the THC and other cannabinoids existing in the cannabis plant. Continue this step for one to two minutes.

4. Filter the crushed cannabis plant using a coffee filter or strainer and transfer the resulting solvent/oil mixture to a separate container. Then set the solvent/oil mixture aside. The above steps have removed around 80% of THC and other cannabinoids from the cannabis plant.

5. Add more solvent to the crushed (and filtered) cannabis plant just sufficient to cover it. Then gently crush the cannabis plant again for another one to two minutes to obtain the remaining THC and other cannabinoids from the plant.

6. Filter the crushed cannabis plant again and transfer the new solvent/oil mixture to the container that holds that first mixture.

7. Throw away the crushed and filtered cannabis plant.

8. Using a coffee filter, form a funnel and put it into the opening of a big clean bottle. Transfer the solvent/oil mixture into the clean bottle through the coffee filter-lined funnel. This helps strain out any residual cannabis plant material. You may repeat this step several times until you feel confident that there are no more residual plant material in the mixture to ensure a good quality and pure cannabis oil.

Warning for the next two steps: DO NOT utilize a heat source with open flame when boiling the solvent, as the fumes from the solvent are extremely flammable. Utmost caution should be practiced in doing steps 9 and 10!

9. Use a rice cooker to boil away the solvent in the mixture. Make sure that the rice cooker is not filled more than ¾ of capacity. Set the rice cooker to "white rice" setting or high heat. As you see the solvent evaporates from the mixture, continue to add the solvent/oil mixture in the rice cooker. When only one inch of the mixture is left in the rice cooker, lift the pot (make sure that you are wearing oven mitts) and lightly swirl the contents. It is important that you work in an outdoor area which is properly ventilated. Turn on the fan to help carry away the fumes from the solvent. Also ensure that your working area is free from cigarettes, sparks and other red-hot elements that can ignite the solvent fumes. It is highly advisable to always wear a face mask to prevent yourself from inhaling the fumes. You also need to ensure that the oil is not heated over 290 degrees F since it can result to the vaporization of the cannabinoids.

10. Do not remove the cannabis oil from the rice cooker unless you are sure that the solvent has completely evaporated. Use oven mitts to hold the rice cooker pot and gently transfer the cannabis into a glass or stainless steel container.

11. Place the container holding the newly prepared cannabis oil on a candle warmer or other gentle heating device to completely evaporate the Co2 from the oil. This process might take several

hours (3 to 10 hours). You will know that the oil is ready for use when you see no more bubbles or activity on the surface of the cannabis oil. The longer amount of time you use in heating the cannabis oil over gentle heat, the more sedative your oil will be. You can also opt to complete the heating process of the oil by placing it in the oven at 230 degrees F for around one hour.

12. To store your newly created cannabis oil, you can use plastic oral syringes that can make it easier for you to take the medicine. But you can also choose to leave the cannabis oil in a stainless container and directly take it from there. Another option is to place the cannabis oil into empty pill capsules so it can be taken in the form of pills.

13. When the cannabis oil is cooled off, its color will become dark brown and its consistency will be similar to heavy grease. But if the oil is thinly spread on a white paper, you will see that its color is actually golden. Some varieties of cannabis plants can produce oil with a very thick consistency, making it difficult to squeeze out of a syringe. If this is the case, you can soften the oil by putting the syringe in warm water a couple of minutes prior to using it.

14. To preserve the freshness of your cannabis oil, ensure that it is stored at room temperature away from humidity and light. It is important that all residual water moisture is evaporated to prevent you cannabis oil from going rancid.

# Chapter 3: Proper Dosage of Cannabis Oil

For majority of people, 60 g/ml of cannabis oil is enough to eradicate most of their cancer cells. On average, it normally takes around ninety days to consume the total amount of 60 g/ml cannabis oil treatment. But you need to recognize that the 60 g/ml and 90 day treatment program is simply a suggestion and a good starting point for treating cancer. Some patients may require more time to consume the full 60 g/ml treatment.

You should begin your cannabis oil treatment by ingesting 3 doses of the oil orally every day. For the 1st week, one dosage is equal to the size of ½ of white rice grain. You can then double the dosage in week 2. After the 2nd week, start doubling the dosage every 4 days until you consume 1 g/ml per day. If you follow the above dosage increase, you will begin to consume 1 g/ml of cannabis oil per day within 30 to 35 days. Once you reach this point, you can maintain this dosage until your cancer is completely gone. However, some patients have been prescribed to increase their daily dosage to 2 g/ml or even more.

Since it is recommended to start taking cannabis oil in small doses, it is ideal to use an oral syringe to fill empty pill capsules. This allows you to be consistent and precise in taking the proper cannabis oil dosage and avoid the "high" side effect of cannabis oil. Using pill capsules will also help you to prepare the treatment dosages weeks or even months in advance and properly monitor how much cannabis oil you are currently consuming. Cannabis oil pills can safely be integrated with other prescribed medications.

It is important that you follow the recommended increase in dosage above, particularly during the first 30 days, to allow your body to slowly build up its tolerance to cannabis oil. If you experience extreme fatigue during the day or the "high" side effect of cannabis oil, it is ideal for you to make a slight reduction in your dosage during daytime and make a corresponding dosage increase before you sleep. This is effective in improving your sleep quality while building your tolerance to cannabis oil during sleep. Keep in mind that different people have varying tolerances for different types of medication.

Your body weight and size are two of the factors that can influence your tolerance to cannabis oil. You also need to be aware that one of the side effects of cannabis oil is that it can lower your blood pressure. If your doctor has prescribed another medication to help in controlling your high blood pressure, you may no longer be required to take them while taking cannabis oil. However, please coordinate closely with your doctor to ensure that you will not experience harmful side effects.

After you have completed the cannabis oil treatment, it is ideal to continue taking the oil at a lower dosage to maintain your health. The recommended dosage is 1 g/ml each month. Some patients who have completed the cannabis oil treatment and have completely stopped taking the oil have experience mild withdrawal symptoms that include lack of sex drive, sweats, loss of appetite and lack of sleep. But you do not have to worry because these withdrawal symptoms normally disappear within seven days.

Large Dose of Cannabis Oil

Patients who require help in getting off dangerous and addictive pain medicines such as Vicodin or Morphine can start taking cannabis oil in large doses. When people addicted to Vicodin or Morphine start taking cannabis oil, they can normally reduce their pain medicines by as much as half. Patients who suffer from late stage cancer, can also benefit from starting their cannabis oil treatment in large doses. But whether you want to start with small or large dose, the important thing is for you to ensure that you stay within your own comfort zone. As I indicated earlier, everyone has a different tolerance to cannabis oil. You need to work closely with your doctor (a doctor who supports the treatment of cancer with cannabis oil) in finding the right dosage for you.

Many testimonials hail the tremendous benefits of cannabis oil and its high success rate in the treatment of cancer. Some people who started their cannabis oil treatment after being seriously harmed by radiation and chemotherapy reported that the amount of time required for the treatment to take effect and kill all cancer cells may take longer.

Depending on the cancer type and extent of damage done, killing the cancer can take as long as six months and as much as 180 g/ml of cannabis oil. But aside from killing the cancer cells, cannabis oil can also aid in rejuvenating vital body organs such as the pancreas. Some patients with diabetes reported that they were able to reduce their insulin intake by half after around 6 weeks of cannabis oil treatment, while other diabetic patients were able to completely stop their insulin intake when their pancreas started to function properly again after the cannabis oil treatment.

Taking cannabis oil for weight loss can be very effective. However, it is important to choose a cannabis strain high in CBD and low in THC. THC is known to increase the appetite, causing "munchies", while CBD suppresses our appetite. Testimonials have reported weight loss of over 30 pounds in five months. When choosing to use cannabis oil for weight loss, please do so responsibly and read Chapter 5 carefully, ensuring a healthy, nutritious diet.

# Chapter 4: Cannabis Oil Treatment for Skin Cancer

In order to ensure successful treatment of skin cancer, you will require around one ounce of high quality cannabis plant to produce three to four grams of high quality cannabis oil. Apply the cannabis oil directly to the skin affected by the cancer and then protect the skin using a hygienic bandage. It is advisable to apply fresh cannabis oil onto the affected skin every day or every other day.

Always use a fresh bandage. Continue the cannabis oil application until all the cancer has disappeared. Once the affected area has healed, continue applying cannabis oil for around two more weeks to ensure that all cancer cells have been eradicated.

If you have been suffering from the skin cancer for a longer period of time, you might need a longer period to completely treat your illness. In the majority of reported skin cancer cases treated with cannabis oil, the cancer normally vanishes within 3 weeks or even less.

Be patient and keep applying the oil until you are fully healed. The amount of time required for your treatment will depend on the severity of your skin cancer and your own rate of healing.

# Chapter 5: Important Lifestyle and Diet Changes

After you have made the decision to start using cannabis oil in treating your cancer or other another illness, it is important for you to know that there are certain lifestyle and diet changes that you need to incorporate in your daily life in order to increase your chances of success. You need to recognize that cancer cells will find it hard to develop in a highly oxygenated and alkaline body. As such, you should start including foods that are rich in alkaline such as green leafy vegetables in your regular diet. Plant protein is also very effective in fighting the development of cancer cells. Chlorophyll has been considered the best alkalizing food so it is ideal to integrate it in your daily diet. Keep in mind that chlorophyll helps plants absorb sunlight and then convert that to usable energy. When you include chlorophyll in your regular diet by eating super greens and dark green leafy vegetables, you are actually eating liquid oxygen. .It is ideal to purchase a juicer, or high quality blender, enabling you to eat large amounts of fruits and vegetables (I highly recommend this juicing book). As much as possible, avoid dairy and meat products since the proteins found in these food products help in promoting the growth of cancer cells. Stop consuming foods rich in sugar and immediately stop drinking any types of soda. Instead of using regular sugar, you can opt to use raw honey, coconut sugar, or other natural sweeteners.

If you smoke, you need to stop it immediately. Smoke from cigarettes continues to kill more than half a million people every year. It has also been scientifically proven that smoking can cause cancer.

Using a juicer, you can make a smoothie composed of 1/3 celery, 1/3 carrot and 1/3 apple and take it every day to increase your Ph level. Eating the seeds of 2 apples on a daily basis can also supply you with the required dosage of B17 which has been known to help in treating various types of cancer.

A lot of people have tried taking cannabis oil as treatment for their cancers but failed to change their lifestyle and diet. In the end, they felt frustrated because the oil was not effective in treating their disease. Keep in mind that changing your regular diet is a matter of life and death. If you want your cancer to be cured, a healthy diet should be your top priority.

Oxygenating your body to help in treating your cancer will be very beneficial. Research studies have shown that most types of cancer resulted from a deficiency of oxygen respiration in the cells of the body. As such, oxygenating your body can prove to be effective in killing the cancer cells. To do this, you can do light bouncing on a 3 feet trampoline for at least twenty minutes every day. This activity can help in oxygenating your body and rapidly increasing your white blood cell count. If you do not have a trampoline, you can simply go out and walk 3 to 4 times every week without fatigue. This will help to increase your oxygen intake.

Lastly, I highly recommend you start drinking non-fluoridated, non-chlorinated spring water on a daily basis. One gallon of this with half a teaspoon of Himalayan pink salt is enough to increase the electricity in your body that is required for rapid healing.

# Conclusion

Thank you again for purchasing this book!

I hope the information provided to you in this book will help you with your healing process. Ultimately it is up to you to take charge, challenge general opinion and listen to your body and intuition. From my own experience, cannabis oil has worked a "miracle" in my family's well-being and ongoing health, which has inspired me to write a compact "how-to" guide on the benefits of cannabis oil. I hope you now have a good understanding of how cannabis oil can cure cancer and how to make your own oil at home.

I am looking forward to receiving your book reviews and feedback on Amazon.com.

Wishing you well!

# Appendix

## Preview of 'GMO Free Diet: The Ultimate Guide on Avoiding GMO Foods and keeping Your Family Healthy with a GMO Free Diet' by Michael Skinner

## Chapter 1- GMOs: The Big No-No!

Genetically Modified Organisms (or GMOs) have swept the world of consumption and biotechnology industry in a very controversial manner. The term itself has prompted several countries to ban their production. Many skeptical consumers have likewise challenged state laws in making GMO labeling mandatory in all food products sold on the market.

*BUT the question is – what really are these so-called GMOs?*

To quote World Health Organization's definition: "GMOs are organisms in which the genetic material (DNA) has been altered in a way that does not occur naturally".

As the name suggests, GMOs are 'genetically engineered' foods or crops. The genetic makeup of these foods is modified or manipulated artificially through validated genetic engineering process. The process has created a range of produce, which are engineered so as to control characteristics such as disease resistance, pesticide resistance, herbicide resistance, nutritional content, and even ripening. Thus, this is a new science that evidently produces 'unstable' bacteria and viruses that could never be produced through natural methods. To put simply, GMOs are 'manipulated' to confer certain traits that are not natural for the organism.

Commercial GMOs have anchored their way on the global market through enticing promises which include:

- Increased yield

- Climate-change ready crops

- Reduced need for the use of pesticides and/or herbicides

- Improved nutrition content of the crops compared to naturally grown produce

- Reduced risks of food shortage

On the other hand, with the growing popularity of GMOs come a range of issues connected to environmental damages and health problems, as well as the violation of farmers' rights and consumer's rights.

## So how did GMOs break into the global market?

The transfer of DNA from one organism to another was found possible and viable back in 1946. However, the real application took place roughly four decades after this discovery. The first ever recorded genetically modified/engineered plant came about in 1983, when a tobacco plant was made anti-biotic resistant.

In 1994, The Food and Drug Administration in the US approved the sale of 'Flavr Savr' tomato, the first food-related genetically modified organism. The company, Calgene in California, started to produce this tomato variant using genetically engineered seeds that have been injected with ACC synthase. Such gene allows ripening to take place after the tomatoes have been picked manually. This particular product has also become a catalyst for the production of more GMOs- particularly the BT corn, BT potato, and canola. Glyphosate (herbicide) –resistant squash followed suit. In 2010, another GMO breakthrough was recorded when scientists were able to augment the Vitamin A content of rice. This rice variant has been on the commercial market ever since.

To read more, please visit Amazon.com.

# Other Book Recommendations:

"Juicing for Health: The Essential Guide To Healing Common Diseases with Proven Juicing Recipes and Staying Healthy For Life" by Donna Cavanaugh

"The Auto Immune Solution: Learn how to Prevent and Overcome Inflammatory Diseases and Live a Pain-Free Life" by Anthony Weil

"Edible Wild Plants for Beginners: The Essential Edible Plants and Recipes to Get Started by Althea Press

"On My Own Two Feet: From Losing My Legs to Learning the Dance of Life" by Amy Purdy

Made in the USA
San Bernardino, CA
05 July 2016